YOUR KNOWLEDGE HAS VALUE

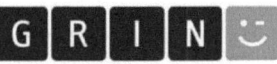

Bibliographic information published by the German National Library:

The German National Library lists this publication in the National Bibliography; detailed bibliographic data are available on the Internet at http://dnb.dnb.de .

Imprint:

Copyright © 2015 GRIN Verlag, Open Publishing GmbH
Print and binding: Books on Demand GmbH, Norderstedt Germany
ISBN: 9783668237551

This book at GRIN:

http://www.grin.com/en/e-book/333873/impact-of-health-behaviour-on-maternal-health-in-bangladesh

Kamalesh Dey

Impact of health behaviour on maternal health in Bangladesh

gladesh

The social, cultural and religious framework

GRIN Publishing

GRIN - Your knowledge has value

Since its foundation in 1998, GRIN has specialized in publishing academic texts by students, college teachers and other academics as e-book and printed book. The website www.grin.com is an ideal platform for presenting term papers, final papers, scientific essays, dissertations and specialist books.

Visit us on the internet:

http://www.grin.com/

http://www.facebook.com/grincom

http://www.twitter.com/grin_com

UNIVERSITY OF BEDFORDSHIRE

FACULTY OF HEALTH AND SOCIAL SCIENCES

MSC PUBLIC HEALTH

HEALTH AND SOCIAL CARE INEQUALITIES

MODULE UNIT CODE: PUB0013-6

ESSAY

ON

IMPACT OF HEALTH BEHAVIOUR ON MATERNAL HEALTH IN
BANGLADESH

JANUARY 2015

WORDS COUNT: 4340

Content

IMPACT OF HEALTH BEHAVIOUR ON MATERNAL HEALTH IN BANGLADESH

INTRODUCTION

The essay will talk about maternal health and health behaviour in Bangladesh. It will also critically explore the actual fact in Bangladesh, how maternal health is influenced by their health behaviour based on social, cultural and religious framework. Moreover, it will also highlight governmental strategy for improving maternal health what will be outstanding achievement of "Millennium Development Goal (MDG) 5" in Bangladesh.

Maternal health is the prime concern of public health in Bangladesh. After that, Bangladesh is highly motivated for achieving "Millennium Development Goal (MDG) 5" for improving maternal health and reducing maternal mortality rate by 75% between the period of 1990 and 2015. However, Bangladesh government is working hard with partnership organisations for achieving MDG goal, while Bangladesh is on track for fulfilling target of MDG 4 and 5 (UN, 2013). Bangladesh government are promoting safe maternity practice and reducing maternal mortality. Already, government has been expanded and promoted existing health services implementing with new policy and services performing EOC (essential obstetric care) services accessible to all women particularly pregnant mothers and adolescent (Anwar et al., 2004)

Moreover, Bangladesh is highly populated developing country in the world with a maternal mortality ratio of 170/100,000 live births (WHO, 2015). Particularly, prenatal and postnatal care is very poor in Bangladesh because of malnutrition. Maximum pregnant mothers are not literate and living with poverty so they are in greater risk during their pregnancy and child birth (BBS, 2013). Walton, Brown and Schbley (2012) stated that in Bangladesh, maternal mortality and morbidity rate is the second highest in the world. There are several influential factors for instances: indigenous health behaviour and traditional lifestyle are remarkable based on social, cultural and religious belief. In Bangladesh, around 20,000 mothers are dying each year during pregnancy period, while 69% (obstetric causes), 14% (injury and violence) and rest 17% deaths indirect causes (Ministry of Health and Family Welfare (MOHFW), 2008).

Almost 99% maternal deaths occur in developing countries, whereas higher than half of the deaths are occurring in sub-Saharan Africa and rest one third occur in South Asia, while rare in developed countries (WHO, 2015). In 2013, maternal mortality ratio was 230 per 100 000 live births in developing countries, while only 16 per 100 000 live births in developed countries. Moreover, the probable number of maternal mortality is only 1 in 3700 in developed countries, while 1 in 160 in developing countries. In 2013, total 289000 women died during their pregnancy period in the world, while almost 800 women are dying only for simple complications during their pregnancy and child birth periods (WHO, 2015).

Royal College of Nursing (2002) stated that determinants of health are the cumulative conditions where people born, grow up, live and work what include accommodation, education, economic status and living environment and health system, while these is variable changed by social and political circumstance.

Moreover, World Health Organisation (WHO, 2015) defined that determinants of health generally depends on particular circumstances include: social and economic status, physical status, and person's individual status (behaviours and characteristics). However, individual's health is absolutely depends on the following factors: Income, education, occupation, social class, gender, race or ethnicity, culture, and religion what play substantial effects on maternal health (Solar and Irwin, 2007).

MATERNAL HEALTH

According to World Health Organisation (WHO) (2014) defined that maternal health is the women's health condition during their whole pregnancy cycle (prenatal, childbirth and postnatal period). Maternal health of any particular country is measured by several parameters for instances: nutritional status (BMI-body mass index), epidemiological report like maternal mortality and morbidity rate and prenatal and postpartum care, contraceptive prevalence rate (CPR), coverage of tetanus toxoid (TT) vaccination, percentage of live bath.

Moreover, maternal health refers to the health of women during pregnancy, childbirth and the postpartum period. In Bangladesh, in minor cases women experience better in their maternity though maximum women are suffering, ill-health and even death. The major direct causes of maternal morbidity and mortality include haemorrhage, infection, high blood pressure, unsafe abortion, and obstructed labour (WHO, 2008).

In addition, in Bangladesh leading cause of maternal mortality is obstetric what leads about 69% maternal death (MOHFW, 2008). Graham et al. (2008) claimed that a woman could be died due to direct or indirect obstetric cause over than 41 days but below one year after pregnancy termination, while direct pregnancy-related death could be defined as: death of women during pregnancy period or termination of pregnancy (not more than 42 days) or other causes is called direct pregnancy death.

In Bangladesh, rural areas due to cultural and religious barrier and lack of education rural women and particularly in slum areas women are accessing maternal health care service as result maternal health situation still in questionable! Most common causes of maternal mortality include postpartum haemorrhage, eclampsia. In addition, domestic violence is also remarkable factors of maternal mortality. In addition, demotic violence (including physical abuse, deprived food, education, care, mental torture) is the remarkable reason what leads about 14% maternal deaths during their pregnancy period(MOHFW, 2015). According to Bangladesh Bureau of statistics (BBS) (2013) reported that in rural Bangladesh, about 22.4% women are victims of physical tortures (beatings), 27% mental torture and rest 34% of verbal abuse where particular young women are more vulnerable under this violence.

Bangladesh is the second highest maternal mortality rate in the world. However, Bangladesh recently, attained considerable improvement of maternal health and reduced maternal mortality rate by expanding promotional health program achieving MDG 5.

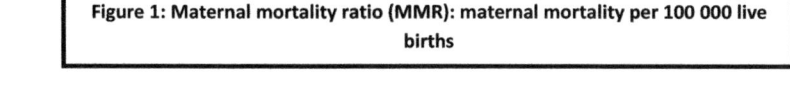

Figure 1: Maternal mortality ratio (MMR): maternal mortality per 100 000 live births

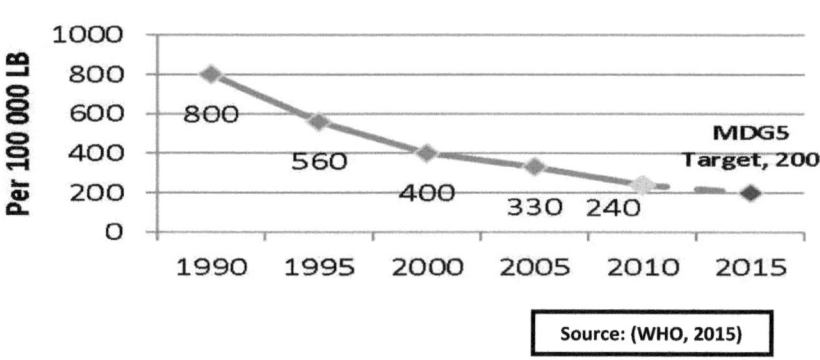

Basically two targets have to fulfil for achieving MDG 5 for instance: reduction of maternal mortality rate by 75% between 1990 and 2015 and accomplishment of universal reproductive health access by 2015 what about to reach (figure 1 and table 1). After implementing government new initiation for achieving MDG 5, maternal mortality rate substantially reduced in 2013 what was 170 per 100 000 live births. In 2001, Maternal Mortality Ratio (MMR) was about 320 per 100 000 live births, while 1990 rate was 570/100,000 live births what almost 44% reduction. Though, that period maximum maternal death occurred at home and Neonatal mortality rate (NMR) was also high as 37 per 1000 live births in 2007 (WHO, 2015).

Table 1: Maternal mortality in 1990-2013

Year	Maternal mortality ratio (MMR)	Maternal deaths	Number of AIDS-related indirect maternal deaths	Live births[a]
	Per 100 000 live births (lb)	Numbers	Numbers	Thousands
2013	170 [94-300]	5,200	1	3,135
2005	260 [150-480]	8,800	0	3,349
2000	340 [190-620]	12,000	0	3,570
1995	440 [240-790]	16,000	0	3,696
1990	550 [310-990]	21,000	0	3,764

Source: (WHO, 2015)

Maternal morbidity is also unacceptable like mortality ratio. Actual rate of morbidity data is impossible as limited number of data is available from Bangladesh demographic health survey. However, mortality and nutritional status is high among women rather than men so it predictable as morbidity rate is also high.

In Bangladesh, girls are more prone affecting iron deficiency anaemia (IDA). Particularly, in rural areas women are more susceptible as the prevalence of IDA about 50 to 90% of pregnant women where 13% women are higher risk making complications during their last pregnancy period (Moran et al., 2009). Moreover, the remarkable complications were abdominal pain (about 25.31%), inflammation of leg or some part of the body (23.33%), IDA (19.94%), urine infections (16.76%), eclampsia (1.99%) and haemorrhage (3.51%). One is every 21 mothers' life is in risk during their pregnancy period (UNICEF, 2009).

Rahman, Parkhurst and Normand (2003) reported that in Bangladesh, about four million women conceive baby yearly but among them about 600,000 women are predictable facing complications during their pregnancy life. About 9 million women developed permanent complications during their pregnancy for instances: fistulae, inability to control urination and painful intercourse what excluded from their family and husband (MOHFW 2008). During pregnancy complications only 21.9% received medical care. Kamal (2012) stated that about 48% women did not receive any medical care during their bleeding. Maximum cases women did not take any care where 61% oedema, 56% vomiting, 35% fever and 19% for high blood pressure. It proved that, in Bangladesh maternal outcomes was so poor, while women were facing complications but they did not seek any care due to their traditional thought and health behaviour.

In addition, according to report only 7.9% child was born in hospital and 5% delivery complications sought out under medical care (Rahman, Parkhurst and Normand, 2003). NIPORT (2001) also reported that only few number of mothers access maternal care through their whole maternity cycle (figure 2).

Figure 2: Selected Maternal Care in Bangladesh

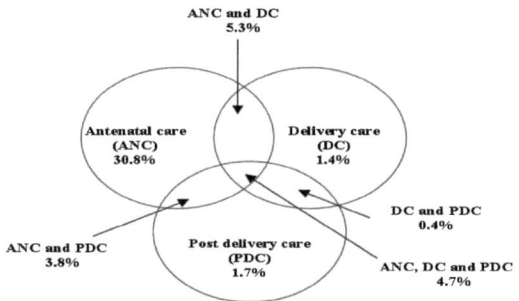

Percentage of births for which mothers received
neither ANC nor DC nor PDC: 51.7 percent

Source: (National Institute of Population Research and Training (NIPORT), 2001)

Moreover, there are many reasons of maternal mortality in Bangladesh where health behaviours are commonly responsible. For instances: high prevalence of anaemia is identified among pregnant women in Bangladesh what leads low birth weight baby as well as create more pregnancy complications; early marriage and adolescent pregnancy also increases the rate of pregnancy complications what influence the maternal and neonatal death (Graham and Hussein, 2006).

In Bangladesh, gender discrimination, lack of education, lack of reproductive knowledge, social, cultural and religious barrier, poverty and poor reproductive care are the main key points of poor maternal what lead high maternal mortality rate (Paul and Rumsey , 2002). Moreover, women are restricted and no possible freedom only for health behaviour, traditional cultural practice and religious barrier, gender discrimination in patriarchy society. Due to underline causes women are not accessing health care particularly in rural community in Bangladesh (Begum, Nili and Sayem, 2010).

Quayyum et al. (2013) stated that social status is the main barrier of maternal health inequalities for instance: poor family always deprived from good maternal care service, while good quality of maternal health service is focused only among rich family. Sometimes poor cannot access health care so rate of maternal mortality is higher in rural areas rather than urban as rich family is living urban area. Moreover, lack of education, cultural and religious barriers, high cost of access and on limited service and lack of skilled care are cumulatively creating inequalities of health care in Bangladesh.

In addition, there is also lack of health care professionals (maternal health specialist, midwives, and nurses) what directly affect maternal health care service. So, lack of skilled health maternal health is performed with poor quality what could make complications. Lack of community based clinic, rural population unable to access health care so poor class who are living village are depriving from the health service (WHO, 2015).

HEALTH BEHAVIOUR

Health behaviour is the individual's characteristics based of health knowledge. Health behaviour is accomplished by health determinants. Conner and Norman (2005, p2) defined that "health behaviour is an activity undertaken by a person believing himself to be healthy for the purpose of preventing disease or detecting it at an asymptomatic stage". Health behaviour is variable what is determined by various factors for examples: social and cultural factors, religious factors and individual's choice. Therefore, health behaviour has significant impact of maternal health in Bangladesh.

Moreover, Health behaviour refers to the intellectual social abilities for controlling inspiration of an individual's ability for understanding the way of development and sustaining good health. Including health education, behaviour oriented communication, political and social factors what determine health. Health behaviour is more widespread comprehensible to stimulate the lifestyle decision and making much more consciousness of the determinants of health what also influence women's reproductive health (WHO, 2015).

Figure3: Determinates of Health

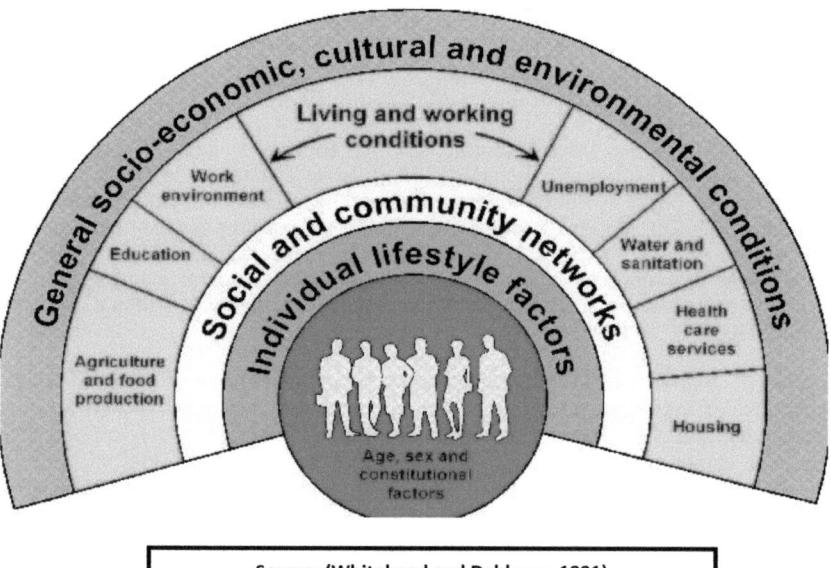

Source: (Whitehead and Dahlgren, 1991)

Royal College of Nursing (2002) stated that health behaviour is modified directly by determinants of health. Determinants of heath are the indicator of individual's health. There are several factors which can measure the actual health status. Socioeconomic factors, cultural factors, religious factors, education, employment, poverty, living condition, housing, individual lifestyles, community networks also determine the health status. These factors also influence the maternal health and reproductive health of women and also accessing to maternal health care services (Whitehead and Dahlgren, 1991).

In Bangladesh, maternal health is fully depends on their health behaviour and individual's belief, traditional culture and religious belief, poverty, education, lack of freedom of women which are the key concern of maternal health as such factors are the hindrance of accessing health care during women's reproductive and pregnancy period.

Education and Freedom

Education is the significant part of woman's life for leading her life healthier. She can gain knowledge through education about their health particularly their reproductive health. Unfortunately, in rural Bangladesh majority of the women are illiterate even 26% were illiterate and they did not go school and 93% are housewives. Nearly, more than half of the mothers get marry before the age of 18 years and 32% mothers age between 18 and 19 years, where 59% mothers conceive baby just before the age of 20 years (Marmot, 2005). Consequently, they have no enough knowledge due to lack of education. Lack of education they are not aware making decision even they have no freedom in patriarchy society. So there are unable to make decision. only, 7 to 10% mothers are able to make decision their maternal care and their health behaviour (food, accommodation, personal likings), 87% mothers are unable to make decision independently but they can make decision with their family and husband (BBS, 2013).

Rahman, Parkhurst and Normand (2003) also reported that about 80% of women did not sick any health facility, 54% women have no confidence for service and rest problem with lack of freedom including: 71.4% women face trouble arranging money for care services, 44% are unable to access health care due to lack of family permission, 49.2% are not getting any one for supporting to go hospital and rest 63.2% have no idea and no knowledge about their problem as where to go for treatment.

Poverty

Poverty is the main problem for accessing health care service. During pregnancy period only few numbers of mothers take full care (antenatal, post natal and delivery care) as In Bangladesh almost majority of the people are living below the poverty line, particularly in rural population of Bangladesh are poor so lack of money they are unable to seek maternal care. NIPORT (2001) reported that only 58% women are unable to afford cost during their pregnancy complications and 24% are able to afford partially, while 35% are unable to afford so they do not seek maternal care even during their complications. They follow normally traditional system and call Dhai (women who act as non-skilled midwives).

Income and social class

Income generally is the most important determinants of socioeconomic position.
Income and social class are directly connected making better maternal health. But the great barrier is the poverty as maximum women living in rural areas are poor rather than urban. In rural Bangladesh, Majority of the family depend on agricultural job so they have poor income and lower social class. Consequently, women living rural areas are more prone making complications during their pregnancy even throughout the maternal life cycle (MOHFW, 2008). In addition, there are less number of skill births attendance in rural areas rather than urban. Anwar et al. (2008) reported that skilled births attendance in urban areas is 42.8%, while in rural areas only 32% though majority of the women are living rural areas so this ratios is too less than urban women.

Occupation

Occupation is the best indicator of individual's health condition as health is correlated with their occupation. It is also specify the socioeconomic status of an individual. Even, occupation replicates the social standard what is related to health outcomes due to some benefits for instances: easy to access for better health care, access of education and good accommodation and better lifestyles(Solar and Irwin, 2007). In Bangladesh, maximum people are doing agricultural job so their social status is low and health status also poor. For the reasons, maternal health is poor lack of accessing maternal care services. In Bangladesh, only17.4% mothers receive full maternal care, while 32% are unable to access health (BBS, 2013)

Culture

Culture is the most important factors in health behaviour what has great role for maintaining individual health. In Bangladesh, people are fully adopted in traditional culture and health behaviour and individual's belief, particularly Women's maternal is commonly emerged with traditional culture and cultural belief.
Reeves and Baden (2000) stated that culture is the unique decorations of an individual thoughts, beliefs, and customs which are symbolised of approach through the lifecycle and relationships with friends, society or groups within a community. Montanari and Sonnenfeld (2006) also indicated that cultural is the intersection between tradition and modernisation. Moreover, culture depends on religion, society, race and ethnicity. Likewise, it is often claimed that culture is learned and shared from one to individuals even other person's value, beliefs, norms and rules of their society. However, culture is also influential for an individual's health as well.

Rahman, Parkhurst and Normand (2003) stated that in Bangladeshi rural culture belief maternal illness is the cause of evil power due to particular food intake or undefined physical causes, while young mothers do not belief like all elder members belief in their family. Consequently, young mothers have to face problem and stay in more restricted way due to ignorance of elder's people advice. Rozario (1995) also mentioned that in rural areas due to traditional cultural belief almost maximum child born at home and unhygienic condition controlled by unqualified Dai (midwives) what leads to high maternal mortality

In addition, women's movements are more restriction during pregnancy and they have no freedom due to social and cultural superstition for instances: going out at night, afternoon and exact noon (12pm) with unfolding hair, going out with unfolding shari or loose dress what might touches on the ground. It is thought to connecting evil power during that specific period in a day. In addition, many food taboos also common during pregnancy period for examples: pineapple (though to cause of abortion), coconuts (making blind baby or white eye), and duck's egg (though to cause asthma of baby), while in some regions hot food is recommended to be avoided. In addition, according to Hindu culture women are not allowed to eat fish and meat for one month, while Muslim women only seven days after delivery (Goodburn, Gazi and Chowdhury, 1995).

Moreover, In Bangladesh, there are 27 deferments types of superstitions which are quite detrimental for accomplishing healthy and safe maternity life cycle Maximum superstitions are related to limiting of the women's movements, intake of proper amount of food what is helpful for the growth of the foetus, while another superstition as eating more is harmful as heavy eating will build up large baby. Besides, there are many harmful social practices still exist particularly in rural areas of Bangladesh what is making complications during pregnancy period for examples: internal manipulation and massage, tight abdominal bands during labour and not using uterine message preventing postpartum haemorrhage (Rahman, Parkhurst and Normand, 2003).

In general, Khan, Grubner and Kramer, (2012) stated that maternal health is more risky in rural areas in Bangladesh where mainly maternal health is influenced by traditional belief as well as lots of misconception about health practice. During traditional birth attendance Dai (Midwives) is the lead person who has basically no training and education. According to evidence, Dai normally use blade without sterilising to cut the umbilical cord and a mixture of burnt earth and cow manure for dressing what is more likely risk of infections (Rozario, 1995).

Paul and Rumsey (2002) also stated that population from rural part of Bangladesh always prefer traditional birth attendance rather than hospital delivery, while traditional birth attendance is highly risk for making pregnancy complications as well as harm for new born baby for examples: mother death, child death, disability, huge bleeding. Bangladesh bureau of statistics (BBS, 2013) reported that only 27% child born in hospital and among that only 11% births in the attendance of health care professionals , while 71% babies born at home with the traditional birth attendance.

Religion

Religion is the most important heath behaviour factor what can influence easily maternal health. In Bangladesh, Muslim 83 -90%, 8-9% Hindu, and 1-2% population are Buddhists and Christians where health behaviour is absolutely depends on their religious view (MOHFW, 2008). Sometimes, religious belief makes people restricted performing any activities what good or may be bad. Moreover, Religious belief makes man more spiritual and kindness. People sometime belief religious superstition plays negative impact on maternal health (Young, 1928).

Leslie and Gupta (1989) purported that in Bangladesh, women are restricted to access health care during their pregnancy period for instance: the Muslim and Hindu women avoid using maternal care service where male health professionals are involving due to only tradition of purdah (Vail). Even, they are not willing to travel hospital as women are not allowed to go hospital particularly some religious family who are highly emerged of religious rules. Moreover, some women have to get permission from their husband. Therefore, Women depend on alternative sources of care what is indigenous medicine or spiritual power what is easily accessible for women.

Paul and Rumsey (2002) also stated in rural areas of Bangladesh women's health are more vulnerable due to insufficient pre-natal care and going to health care centre during only emergency condition what is obvious harm for both mothers and child. Even, due to religious restriction Muslim women are less likely access health care centre as doctors, nurses, and staffs are normally unknown. In addition, they feel embarrass to talk and share their problem, hence they prefer traditional birth attendance, consequently, they are more prone of affecting pregnancy complication and predicted high number of maternal mortality only for religious barrier(Rahman, Parkhurst and Normand, 2003).

Paul and Rumsey (2002) also stated that witnessed that in Bangladesh, particularly in rural areas people believe childbirth is a natural process and it is act as gift of God. Even, they prefer traditional birth attendance at home rather than in hospital. Sometimes, illiterate rural people are misguided through blind religious belief. Both Muslim and Hindu women are almost same as they are not willing to take maternal care during pregnancy period.

Schbley (2012) also reported that Muslim women normally get marry at early age in their life about 13.5 years and conceive baby first year of their marriage and have delivery, while Hindu religion does not support early marriage. Moreover, Hindu women are more conscious than Muslim women and they seek their maternal care periodically. The number of skilled birth attendance is higher among Hindu women (61.3%) rather than Muslim women (33.6%), consequently maternal mortality rate is more evident in Muslim family rather than Hindu in Bangladesh (Anwar et al., 2008).

Access and Utilisation of Maternal Health in Bangladesh

In Bangladesh, access and utilisation of maternal health is very poor due to above mentioned factors which is closely related to seeking maternal care. Particularly, rural women are not using health care due to underlying causes for instances: cultural, religious, poverty. Rahman, Parkhurst and Normand (2003) reported that only 20% women are accessing maternal care during their pregnancy period.

Majority of the mother are not using any anti-natal care, while half of women took medical care during complication of their full pregnancy period and one fifth among them admitted due to abortion and rest of the women admitted for care due to haemorrhage, pre-eclampsia, and mal-presentation and even they are facing lots of problem just before accessing health care (figure 4). Moreover, 56 % women seek health care during pregnancy complications, while 30% women are not getting full facility and only 26% women get full facility during their life threatening (NIPORT, 2001).

Figure 4: Problems in Accessing Health Care

Problems in Accessing Health Care

Category	Percent
Getting someone to accompany	49.2
Getting money needed	71.4
Getting permission to go	44
Lack of confidence in source of service	54.2
Going to health facility	49.6
Health facility far away	79
Knowing where to go	63.2

Percent of mothers

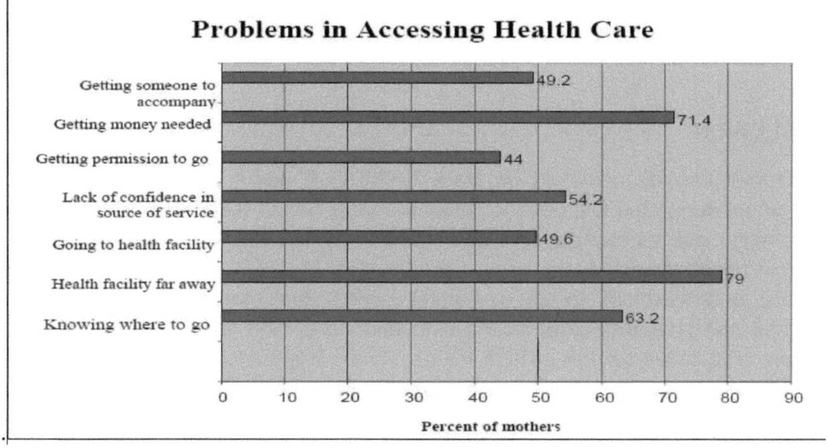

Source: (National Institute of Population Research and Training (NIPORT), 2001)

GOVERNMENT INTERVENTIONS

Maternal health is so poor in Bangladesh, while government are trying to achieve Millennium Development Goal (MDG) 5 reducing the maternal mortality and improving the maternal health. Already government has implemented some extra program, however still maternal health is not improving greatly due to their health behaviour as it's fully adopted on their cultural, religious and social economic factors. So, government initiated the following maternal health strategy for addressing this issue where some of special department are involved to run this initiative. For examples: Human Resource Development (HRD) and Quality Assurance (QA), Behaviour Change Communication (BCC), and Community Participation Program (CPP). According to Bangladesh Ministry of Health and Family (MOHFW), 2008) "The key objects of the Behaviour Change Communication (BCC) are:

➢ Modifying attitude and changing health behaviour among women (especially, living in rural areas) to improve their health and reproductive health condition.
➢ Constructing effective community support for enhancing health seeking behaviour.
➢ Modifying attitude and service provider of health behaviour providing services based on customer's demand.

13

> Encouraging show the respect of men for women and girls in the specific circumstances in the society"

In addition, in micro level the following effective strategy has been edited by government for improving nutritional status of women.

> Eradication of poverty policies, particularly, intended for reducing income and social inequalities.
> Approaches to make availability of safe drinking water and good hygiene and sanitation.
> Approaches to improve food security, particularly among the slum in urban and rural areas.
> Establishment new approaches for nutrition intervention program through nutrition education campaign (MOHFW, 2008).

CONCLUSION

Bangladesh already achieved on track of MDG 5 due to continuous efforts of government during the last decade, while maternal health is still poor in Bangladesh due to high maternal mortality rate as maternal mortality ratio is the ideal indicator of maternal health. Bangladeshi women are living at high risk especially for maternal mortality and morbidity in the postnatal period. Malnutrition, anaemia, lack of antenatal and postnatal care, skilled birth attendants and limited access of health care are cumulative causes of high maternal rate where mostly health behaviour is responsible for seeking less heath care facilities particularly in rural areas in Bangladesh. Generally, maternal health is determined by women's health behaviour and Health behaviour is influenced by culture, religion and socioeconomic factors. These factors are mainly problematic issue leading poor maternal health in Bangladesh. So, maternal health care strategy in Bangladesh ought to be oriented with the nature of culture and religious view improving their health behaviour. Consequently, people's mind could be come out from the cultural and religious barrier. Therefore, their health behaviour could be improved what ultimately develop maternal health status in Bangladesh.

REFERENCES

Anwar, A.T.M.I., Killewo, J., Chowdhury, M.-.K. and Dasgupta, S.K. (2004) 'Bangladesh : Inequalities in utilization of maternal health care services, evidence from MATLAB', [online]. Available at: https://openknowledge.worldbank.org/bitstream/handle/10986/13672/304720RPP2B angladesh.pdf?sequence=1 (Accessed: 20 January 2015).

Anwar, I., Sami, M., Akhtar, N., Chowdhury, M., Salma, U., Rahman, M. and Koblinsky, M. (2008) 'Inequity in maternal health-care services: Evidence from home-based skilled-birth-attendant programs in Bangladesh', *Bulletin of the World Health Organization,* 86 (4), pp.252-259 [online]. Available at: http://www.scielosp.org/pdf/bwho/v86n4/v86n4a09.pdf (Accessed: 19 January 2015).

Bangladesh Bureau of Statistics (BBS) (2013) *'Child and mother nutrition survey' 2012* [online]. Available at: http://www.bbs.gov.bd/WebTestApplication/userfiles/Image/Health_Demo/CMNS.pdf (Accessed: 26 January 2015).

Begum, H.A., Nili, N.Y. and Sayem, A.M. (2010) 'Utilization of maternal health care services in slum areas of Dhaka city, Bangladesh', *Ibrahim Medical College Journal,* 4 (2), pp.44-48 [online]. Available at: http://www.banglajol.info/index.php/IMCJ/article/view/6495/4981 (Accessed: 20 january 2015).

Conner, M. and Norman, P. (2005) *Predicting health behaviour.* Second edn. England: McGraw-Hill International.

Goodburn, E.A., Gazi, R. and Chowdhury, M. (1995) 'Beliefs and practices regarding delivery and postpartum maternal morbidity in rural Bangladesh ', Studies in Family Planning, 26 (1), pp.22-32.

Graham, W.J., Ahmed, S., Stanton, C., Abou-Zahr, C. and Campbell, O.M. (2008) 'measuring maternal mortality: An overview of opportunities and options for developing countries', *BMC Medicine,* 6 pp.12-7015-6-12 [online]. Available at: http://www.biomedcentral.com/content/pdf/1741-7015-6-12.pdf (Accessed: 25 January 20125).

Graham, W.J., Foster, L.B., Davidson, L., Hauke, E. and Campbell, O.M.R. (2008) 'Measuring progress in reducing maternal mortality', *Best Practice and Research Clinical Obstetrics and Gynaecology,* 22 (3), pp.425-445 [online]. Available at: http://ac.els-cdn.com/S1521693407001897/1-s2.0-S1521693407001897-main.pdf?_tid=088d4e0e-a49c-11e4-bc87-00000aab0f26&acdnat=1422195259_8a479c5dc67b3293ffba0a8001d9abfd (Accessed: 21 January 2015)

Kamal, S.M.M. (2012) 'Safe motherhood practices among women of urban slums in bangladesh', *Health Care for Women International,* 33 (8), pp.719-738 [online]. Available at: http://0-eds.b.ebscohost.com.brum.beds.ac.uk/eds/pdfviewer/pdfviewer?sid=7b7500d4-b2a2-47c8-b773-85673c110c04%40sessionmgr198&vid=1&hid=104 (Accessed: 20 january 2015)

Khan, M.M., Grubner, O. and Kramer, A. (2012) 'Frequently used healthcare services in urban slums of Dhaka and adjacent rural areas and their determinants', *Journal of Public Health (Oxford, England),* 34 (2), pp.261-271 [online]. Available at: http://jpubhealth.oxfordjournals.org/content/34/2/261.full.pdf (Accessed: 19 January 2015).

Leslie, J. and Gupta, G.R. (1989) Utilization of formal services for maternal nutrition and health care. International Center for Research on Women Washington, DC.

Marmot, M. (2005) 'Social determinants of health inequalities', *The Lancet,* 365 (9464), pp.1099-1104 [online]. Available at: http://ac.els-cdn.com/S0140673605711466/1-s2.0-S0140673605711466-main.pdf?_tid=53cad354-a574-11e4-a9f6-00000aab0f26&acdnat=1422288156_1ea096bef3f7dd5027b1a4d749438a93 (Accessed: 21 January 2015).

Ministry of Health and Family Welfare (MOHFW) (2008) *Maternal Health Review.* Available at: http://www.mohfw.gov.bd/ (Accessed: 26 January 2015).

Montanari, M. and Sonnenfeld, A. (2006) Food is culture New York: Columbia University Press.

Moran, A.C. (2006) *Maternal Morbidity in Rural Bangladesh: Women's Perceptions and Care Seeking Behaviors, [online].* Available at: https://jscholarship.library.jhu.edu/handle/1774.2/868 (Accessed: 21 January 2015).

National Institute of Population Research and Training (NIPORT) (2001) 'Bangladesh maternal health services and maternal mortality survey 2001', Available at: http://dhsprogram.com/pubs/pdf/OD21/BMMSDIST.pdf (Accessed: 21 January 2015).

Paul, B.K. and Rumsey, D.J. (2002) 'Utilization of health facilities and trained birth attendants for childbirth in rural Bangladesh: An empirical study', Social Science and Medicine, 54 (12), pp.1755-1765 [online]. Available at: http://www.sciencedirect.com/science/article/pii/S0277953601001484# (Accessed: 01 December 2014).

Quayyum, Z., Khan, M.N., Quayyum, T., Nasreen, H.E., Chowdhury, M. and Ensor, T. (2013) '"Can community level interventions have an impact on equity and utilization of maternal health care" - evidence from rural Bangladesh', *International Journal for Equity in Health,* 12 pp.22-9276-12-22 [online]. Available at:

http://www.biomedcentral.com/content/pdf/1475-9276-12-22.pdf (Accessed: 21 January 2015).

Rahman, S.A., Parkhurst, J.O. and Normand, C. (2003) 'Maternal health review Bangladesh', *Policy Research Unit Ministry of Health and Family Welfare Bangladesh,* [online] .Available at: http://diningforwomen.org/wp-content/uploads/2014/04/02-03_bangladesh.pdf(Accessed: 21 January 2015).

Rahman, S.A., Parkhurst, J.O. and Normand, C. (2003) 'Maternal health review bangladesh', Policy Research Unit Ministry of Health and Family Welfare Bangladesh, [online]. Available at: http://r4d.dfid.gov.uk/pdf/outputs/healthsysdev_kp/02-03_bangladesh.pdf (Accessed 01 December 2014)..

Reeves, H. and Baden, S. (February 2000) Gender and developmentconcepts and definitions Los Angeles, Calif; Bridge.

Royal College of Nursing (2002) *Health inequalities and the social determinants of health.* Available at: http://www.rcn.org.uk/__data/assets/pdf_file/0007/438838/01.12_Health_inequalities_and_the_social_determinants_of_health.pdf (Accessed: 26 January 2015).

Rozario, S. (1995) 'Traditional birth attendants in Bangladeshi villages: Cultural and sociologic factors', International Journal of Gynaecology and Obstetrics, 50 pp.S145-S152 [online]. Available at: http://ac.els-cdn.com/0020729295025035/1-s2.0-0020729295025035-main.pdf?_tid=8b6a3ff6-7c85-11e4-93ff-00000aab0f02&acdnat=1417787554_845292509c5ce810662cdb5ab807515c (Accessed 01 December 2014)..

Solar, O. and Irwin, A. (2007) 'A conceptual framework for action on the social determinants of health.' [online]., Available at: http://whqlibdoc.who.int/publications/2010/9789241500852_eng.pdf (Accessed: 21 January 2015).

United Nations (UN) (2013) *'United Nations Millennium Development Goals 5'.* Available at: http://www.un.org/millenniumgoals/pdf/Goal_5_fs.pdf (Accessed: 26 January 2015).

United Nations International Children's Emergency Fund (UNICEF) (2009) *Maternal and neonatal health in Bangladesh.* Available at: http://www.unicef.org/bangladesh/Maternal_and_Neonatal_Health.pdf (Accessed: 25 January 2015).

Walton, L., Brown, D. and Schbley, B. (2012) 'Cultural barriers to maternal health care in rural Bangladesh', Journal of Health Ethics, fall, [online]. Available at: http://papers.ssrn.com/sol3/papers.cfm?abstract_id=2042694 (Accessed 01 December 2014).

Walton, L., Brown, D. and Schbley, B. (2012) 'Cultural barriers to maternal health care in rural Bangladesh', *Journal of Health Ethics, Fall,* 9 (1), [online]. Available at: http://papers.ssrn.com/sol3/papers.cfm?abstract_id=2042694 (Accessed: 21 January 2015)

Whitehead, M. and Dahlgren, G. (1991) 'What can be done about inequalities in health?', *The Lancet,* 338 (8774), pp.1059-1063.

World Health Organisation (WHO) (2014) 'Definition of maternal health'. Available at: http://www.who.int/topics/maternal_health/en/ (Accessed 01 December 2014)..

World Health Organisation (WHO) (2014) 'Maternal Mortality Info graphic'. Available at:http://www.who.int/reproductivehealth/publications/monitoring/maternal-mortality-infographic.pdf?ua=1 (Accessed 01 December 2014).

World Health Organisation (WHO) (2015) *'Health literacy and health behaviour'.* Available at: http://www.who.int/healthpromotion/conferences/7gchp/track2/en/ (Accessed: 26 January 2015).

World Health Organisation (WHO) (2015) *Improving maternal newborn and child health in Bangladesh.* Available at: http://unpan1.un.org/intradoc/groups/public/documents/APCITY/UNPAN022523.pdf (Accessed: 25 January 2015).

World Health Organisation (WHO) (2015) *The determinants of health.* Available at: http://www.who.int/hia/evidence/doh/en/ (Accessed: 1/26/2015).

World Health Organisation (WHO) Bangladesh (2015) *Maternal and neonatal health.* Available at: http://www.searo.who.int/bangladesh/areas/maternal_and_neonatal/en/ (Accessed: 25 January 2015).

World Health Organisation (WHO) Bangladesh (2015) *SEARO | WHO country cooperation strategy Bangladesh 2014–2017.* Available at: http://www.searo.who.int/bangladesh/publications/ccs_ban_2008-2013.pdf (Accessed: 25 January 2015).

World Health Organization (WHO) (2015) *maternal health profile.* Available at: http://www.who.int/maternal_child_adolescent/epidemiology/profiles/maternal/bgd.pf (Accessed: 26 January 2015).

World Health Organization (WHO) (2015) *maternal mortality ratio (global health observatory data repository).* Available at: http://apps.who.int/gho/data/view.main.1390 (Accessed: 26 January 2015).

Young, L.J. (1928) 'What is religion?', Social Science, pp.138-145.

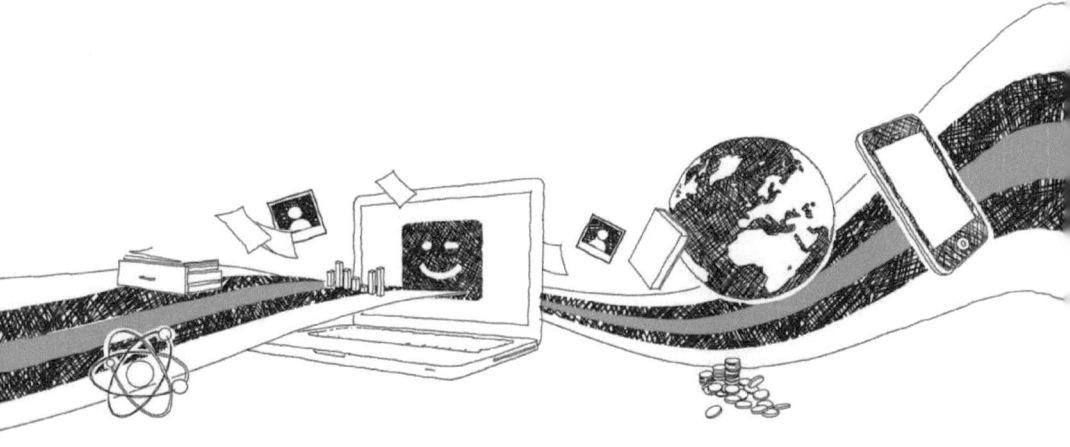
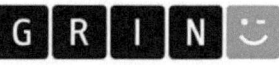